The Teal Survivor

"Beating The Odds"

By: Sue Vernon (Author)

Disclaimer:

 The information provided within this eBook is for general informational purposes only. While we try to keep the information up-to-date and correct, there are no representations or warranties, express or implied, about the completeness, accuracy, reliability, suitability, or availability with respect to the information, products, services, or related graphics contained in this eBook for any purpose. Any use of this information is at your own risk. All pictures contained in this book solely belongs to the Author Sue Vernon. All pictures provided by Sue Vernon are only used for the purposes of this book. No one else has permission to use any or all of the pictures with the sole permission of Author Sue Vernon.

Dedication

Thank you to all my friends, family and even strangers for all your love, prayers and support. I could not have had went through this journey without you. This book is also being dedicated to my aunt Kathy. She passed away at the age 17 from Cervical Cancer.

Preface

Along with numerous Teal sisters, I am
dedicated to helping raise awareness for all
women's cancer (GYN Cancers). I hope that my
story of surviving Cervical Cancer will inspire
you. Cancer is so bad it's almost like it's
contagious. In hopes of writing my story, I hope
that all women at any age will have their
screenings and physicals done every year.
Myself dreaded the physical, but I'm also
thankful today that I went. That one visit to my
OBGYN Doctor, saved my life. That one visit to
my OBGYN Doctor, saved my life. You will be
thankful in the long run that you went.

Table of Contents

Chapter 1

Precancerous At 10

When I was a child, I was just as healthy as my brother, sister, and cousins. I always played, and had a normal life just like every child my age. My grandmother raised me and my siblings along with two of my cousins. She was just like our second mother.

For three years, straight when I was in Elementary School, I received the "Perfect Attendance Award". My grandmother made sure we all went to school. We just about had to have the flu to stay out.

My mother always worked and several times she had to pull double shifts. So, if she was at home, she would sleep from where she was to tired from working.

The day would soon be coming that we never expected to receive the news that we did. I went to my Doctor for a physical. A few days passed and we all wasn't thinking anything of my visit because I had always been healthy. We had no reason to think different.

One afternoon my grandmother received a phone call from the Doctor. He told my grandmother that he was going to have to schedule me for "Laser Surgery" because I had over 1000 precancerous cells on my Cervix. This was a very huge shock. I became scared and afraid. I was only 10 years old and still had my whole life ahead of me.

On the day of my surgery I had no clue what was ahead of me. I was too young to even understand what the older ones were saying. Let alone the doctor using words I never heard of. After I arrive and get checked in to the Hospital, it wasn't long after the nurses came to take me to the Operating Room.

As I returned to my regular room, their stood my mother and my grandmother. I was released he same day a few hours later. I was so glad to go home and no longer have the pre-cancer cells. Even though they were precancerous, they could've either went away, or turned into the main cancer.

When I went for my follow-up with my Doctor two weeks later, I remember him telling me to always make sure I have my regular physicals. The Doctor told me that the pre-cancer cells could come back years later down the road, and could be worse.

I am here today to help encourage women of all ages to have your yearly physicals. Just one Doctor visit can help save your life. Encourage your family and friends to do the same thing. They will thank you in the long run.

Chapter 2

Living With HPV

HPV is the most common sexually transmitted infection. HPV is a different virus than (herpes). HPV is so common that nearly all sexually active people get it at some point in their lives. There are many different types of HPV. Some types can cause health problems including Cervical Cancer. There are vaccines that can stop these health problems from happening.

The Human Papillomavirus Vaccination is given in three different doses. Although all three doses aren't given at the same time.

Both of my daughters at this time, have had their first vaccination. My daughters are eleven years old and fourteen years old. They will go every other two months to get their final two doses.

The reason I had my daughters protected is not only because Cervical cancer runs through the family. But you may never know when something may happen. Such as rape.

Males also can carry this deadly virus. The virus is then passed to the female. It is also recommended for males to get the vaccination just as much as the female.

Chapter 3

Fighting Cervical Cancer

Earlier, I talked about me having precancerous cells at the age of ten. My doctor at that time told me that the cancer cells could return later in life. I never thought of it no more after that, until the real cancer discovered my body.

In June 2016 when I went to have a physical, the test came back abnormal. I was sent to have several biopsies completed.

My OBGYN doctor called and my husband heard the voicemail before I did. With a huge fear that came over him, my husband already knew something was wrong.

The doctor said, "I need you to get to my office as soon as you can". At that time, we didn't know who was more frightened. My husband, the doctor, or myself.

We immediately left to go to the doctor's office. As I approached the front desk, they didn't check me in. The nurse then called me to the back. At that time the doctor came in, and that's when she went over my test results. It was then that I started losing hope. The doctor told me I had the real cancer in my cervix.

The doctor sent me to an OBGYN Oncologist (women's cancer doctor). From there I underwent so much bloodwork, and a even had to have a PETSCAN. A PETSCAN was done to make sure that the cancer wasn't spreading. The cancer doctor said I had a Stage 1B1 Cervical Cancer. Thanks to God above and the good doctors that was treating me, the cancer didn't spread and the caught it just in time.

On September 19, 2016, I underwent a Radical Hysterectomy. The surgery was only supposed to last for up to four hours and lasted six. I was only supposed to have three incisions and had five. My hospital stay was just over night, and I had to wear a catheter for a week. I was so glad when I went for my follow-up. That catheter was very uncomfortable.

I am now cancer free and didn't have no chemo or radiation treatments. My husband, some of my family and friends were very supportive throughout the journey.

My personal advice to all women, is to have your annual check-ups. Even if you are feeling great and no symptoms. Women's cancers are a silent killer. In some cases, you may not have any symptoms until the cancer has gone too far. My family needed me. I done everything that I was supposed to do. That one visit to the doctor saved my life and it can yours to.

My cancer is gone, but I still have to follow-up with my Oncologist every three months. I still dread these visits. Fear could possibly never leave. As I have mentioned before, just one visit can save your life.

Chapter 4

Teal Awareness

The following information on this page have been provided by the Organizations listed. Sue Vernon is only providing this page for informational use and raising awareness.

According to Cancer Treatment Centers Of America, Cervical Cancer begins in the cervix. The Cervix is a narrow organ at the bottom of the uterus that connects to the vagina. The cervix dilates during childbirth to allow for passage of a baby.

Information received from Gardasil.9 Anal cancer affects both males and females. Anal cancer rates have been increasing among Americans. It's believed that about 85% to 90% of anal cancer cases are caused by HPV. And, of those cancers, 90% are caused by seven types. HPV can also lead to vaginal and vulvar cancer.

(HPV= Human Papillomavirus)

Gardasil.9 also stated "not all cases of vaginal, vulvar, and anal cancer are caused by HPV". Approximately 70% to 75% of vaginal cancer cases, 30% of vulvar cancer cases, and 85% to 90% of anal cancer cases are HPV related.
(HPV= Human Papillomavirus)

Chapter 5

Cancer Survivor

As a survivor to Cervical Cancer, I truly hope that my book "The Teal Survivor" has been inspiring to many. My heart goes out to everyone that has fought the battle, and to the very many that are fighting the battle today.

Cancer is a disease that nobody wants and can be deadly if not treated or detected early. Help us spread awareness by encouraging your family and friends to go for a physical. Get your daughters vaccinated to help protect them against the Human Papillomavirus (HPV).

I have heard so many people say that cancer is not genetic. According to the National Cancer Institute, Cancer is a genetic disease. Cancer is caused by certain changes to genes that control the way our cells function, especially how they grow and divide.

According to the National Cancer Institute Genetic changes that promote cancer can be inherited from our parents if the changes are present in germ cells, which are the reproductive cells of the body (eggs and sperm).

Such changes, called germline changes, are found in every cell of the offspring. Genetic tests can tell whether a person from a family that shows signs of such a syndrome has one of these mutations. These tests can also show whether family members without obvious disease have inherited the same mutation as a family member who carries a cancer-associated mutation.

My aunt passed away in 1983 due to Cervical Cancer. I had a father that passed away in 2007 due to complications of Liver Cancer. My sister had Cervical Cancer around 2004. Cancer is a very serious disease and can be deadly at a certain point.

Reference: www.cancercenter.com

The Women's Cancer Resource Center has a lot of valuable information. Please visit their site at www.wcrc.org

Chapter 6

Raising Awareness

The following information is an outline of women's cancer months. Not all cancer or months listed.

February is National Cancer Prevention

September is Gynecologic Cancer Awareness

January is Cervical Cancer Awareness

I encourage everyone to view the awareness calendars to view their complete details.

Wondering how you can help raise awareness? Here's how. Write or share social media posts about recognizing the symptoms of gynecologic cancers and the importance of being treated by a gynecologic oncologist if diagnosed, conduct a Community Event. Ask family members, friends, co-worker's, fellow church goers, to help you spread the word about women's cancers and how fatal the cancer can be. Encourage all females to have a yearly physical.

You may also conduct an online search for more ways to raise and spread awareness.

"Be someone's hero"

Reference:

HPV= Human Papillomavirus

OB/GYN= Obstetrics Gynecology

OB/GYN Oncologist= Cancer Doctor for Women

"Remain Cancer Free"

Chapter 7

Photos By Sue

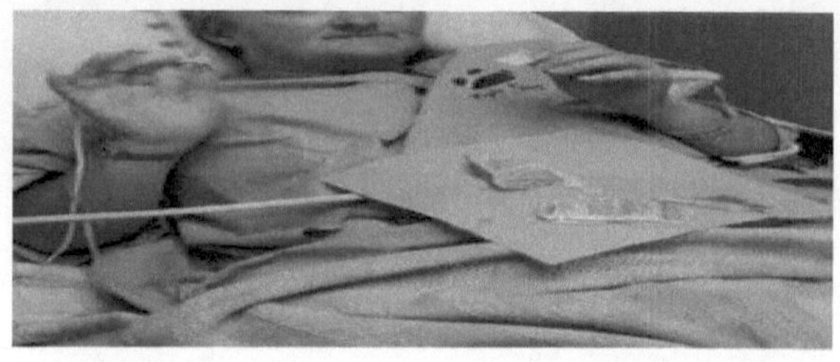

Sue when she had her first biopsy done. Three days later when the test results came back showing she had Cervical Cancer. (June 2016)

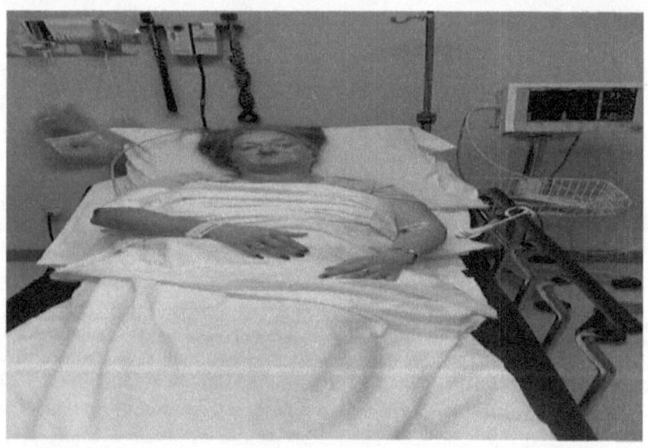

Sue had to visit the hospital. She was having complications from the Cervical Cancer. (July 2016)

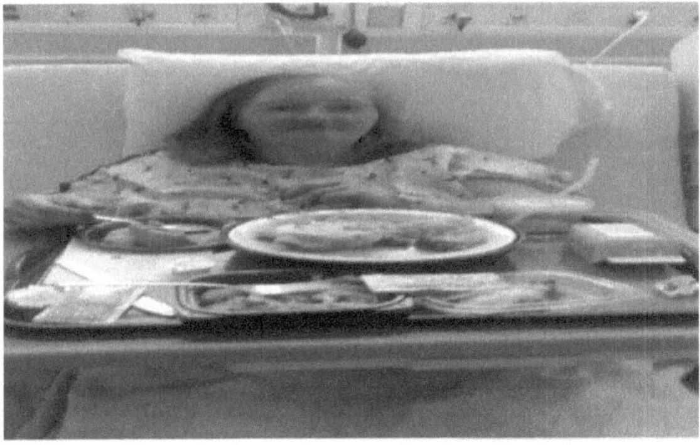

Surgery Day! Sue trying to eat, just hours after her having a Radical Hysterectomy for Cervical Cancer. (September 19, 2016)

Meet The Author

Born and raised in Virginia, Sue loves life. She is a mother of four children (two boys and two girls). Sue is married to the love of her life for almost 11 years.

Sue has worked in the Small Business Industry for more than 13 years. She has been in the cleaning business, and several Direct Sales business.

With so many struggles that faces Sue and her family, it was to the point of her giving up. Sue decided one day that no matter what life threw at her, she had to get all of the stress and anxiety off of her.

Sue Vernon is now writing books not only to help her come out of darkness, but hoping to inspire others. "Sue's Journey" is the first book that Sue has written. The book is non-fiction. All of Sue's stories are based on real life events that she faced.

Sue Vernon   The Teal Survivor

All pictures contained in this book solely belongs to the
Author Sue Vernon. All pictures provided by Sue Vernon
are only used for the purposes of this book. No one else
has permission to use any or all of the pictures with the
sole permission of Author Sue Vernon.